Liu Zi Jue

in the same series

Ba Duan Jin
Eight-section Qigong
Compiled by the Chinese Health Qigong Association
978 1 84819 005 4

Wu Qin Xi
Five-Animal Qigong Exercises
Compiled by the Chinese Health Qigong Association
978 1 84819 007 8

Yi Jin Jing
Tendon–Muscle Strengthening Qigong Exercises
Compiled by the Chinese Health Qigong Association
978 1 84819 008 5

Chinese Health Qigong

Liu Zi Jue

Six Sounds Approach to Qigong Breathing Exercises

Compiled by the Chinese Health Qigong Association

SINGING DRAGON
London and Philadelphia

First published in the United Kingdom in 2008 by
Singing Dragon
An imprint of Jessica Kingsley Publishers
116 Pentonville Road
London N1 9JB, UK
and
400 Market Street, Suite 400
Philadelphia, PA 19106, USA

www.jkp.com

First published in China in 2007 by Foreign Languages Press
24 Baiwanzhuang Road, Beijing, China

Copyright © Foreign Languages Press 2007

Library of Congress Cataloging in Publication Data
Liu zi jue : six sounds approach to qigong breathing exercises / compiled by the Chinese Health Qigong Association.
    p. cm.
  ISBN 978-1-84819-006-1 (pb : alk. paper)
  1. Qi gong. 2. Breathing exercises. I. Zhongguo jian shen qi gong xie hui.
  RA781.8.L5874 2008
  613.7'1489—dc22

                                                           2008014395

British Library Cataloguing in Publication Data
A CIP catalogue record for this book is available from the British Library

ISBN 978 1 84819 006 1

Disclaimer
This book is for reference and informational purposes only and is in no way intended as medical counseling or medical advice. The information contained herein should not be used to treat, diagnose or prevent any disease or medical condition without the advice of a competent medical professional. The activities, physical or otherwise, described herein for informational purposes, may be too strenuous or dangerous for some people and the reader should consult a physician before engaging in them. The author and Singing Dragon shall have neither liability nor responsibility to any person or entity with respect to any loss, damage, or injury caused or alleged to be caused directly or indirectly by the information contained in this book.

Printed and bound by
Reliance Printing (shenzhen)., Ltd, Hong Kong

Contents

Chapter I   Origins and Development   10

Chapter II   Characteristics   13

Chapter III   Practice Tips   17

Chapter IV   Step-by-Step Descriptions of the Routines . .   21

   Ready Position   22

   Starting Position   23

      XU Exercise (嘘字诀)   28

      HE Exercise (呵字诀)   33

      HU Exercise (呼字诀)   43

      SI Exercise (呬字诀)   47

CHUI Exercise (吹字诀)   57

XI Exercise (嘻字诀)   67

Closing Form   75

APPENDIX: ACUPUNCTURE POINTS
MENTIONED IN THIS BOOK   77

Preface

L iu Zi Jue, or Six Sounds Approach to Breathing Exercises, is a traditional health and fitness practice focused on control of the breath. It is part of the *Chinese Health Qigong Exercise Series* compiled by the Chinese Health Qigong Association.

Liu Zi Jue regulates and controls the rise and fall of Qi (vital energy) inside the body and related inhalation and exhalation through different mouth shapes—six in all—to breathe and pronounce the "XU, HE, HU, SI, CHUI, and XI" exercises. As these exercises strengthen the liver, heart, spleen, lungs, kidneys and Sanjiao (the three parts of the body cavities housing the internal organs), respectively, Liu Zi Jue helps to balance the energy and the functions of the inner organs.

These exercises feature slow, gentle, extended and graceful movements. Easy to learn and practice, safe and reliable, they are suitable for people of all ages and conditions of health.

Surveys show that practitioners find that the Liu Zi Jue exercises are easy and graceful. Moreover, a general improvement of the quality of life is reported by those interviewed. Improvement of social relations, especially the lubrication of relationships and decrease of family frictions rank top among the beneficial effects of these exercises. It is believed that this is the result of the gentle breathing movements, which calm the feelings and emotions. Studies and medical tests also note that the exercises are safe, reliable and free from side effects, and help to cure such chronic diseases as hypertension, hyperlipidemia and high blood sugar.

Chapter I

Origins and Development

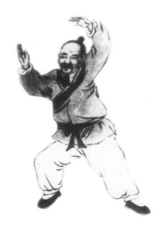

The term Liu Zi Jue first appears in a book called *On Caring for the Health of the Mind and Prolonging the Life Span* (养性延命录),written by Tao Hongjing of the Southern and Northern Dynasties (420–589). A leading figure of the Maoshan School of Taoism, Tao was renowned for his profound knowledge of traditional Chinese medicine. "One has only one way for inhalation, but six for exhalation—CHUI, HU, XI, HE, XU and SI. CHUI gets rid of heat; HU sweeps away wind; XI eliminates worries; HE promotes the circulation of energy; XU drives away cold; and SI reduces stress," he writes in the book. He explains further: "Those with heart disease should practice CHUI, and HU, to drive away cold and heat. Those with lung disease should practice XU, to relieve swelling. Those who have spleen trouble should practice XI, to eliminate stress. As for those who suffer from a liver disease, HE will help to cure it."

Zou Pu'an, of the Song Dynasty (960–1279), was a major contributor, in terms of theory and practice, to the transmission of the exercises. In his book titled *The Supreme Knack for*

Health Preservation—Six-Character Approach to Breathing Exercises (太上玉轴六字气诀), he recommends, "Don't listen to anything when pronouncing the sounds. Close your mouth, lower your head after finishing, breath in fresh air from the universe slowly through the nose. Don't listen to anything when inhaling." He also recommends such preparatory movements as tapping the teeth, licking the front of the teeth with the lips closed and swallowing saliva.

No body movements accompanied the Liu Zi Jue exercises until the Ming Dynasty (1368–1644), when Hu Wenhuan and Gao Lian wrote books on the subject. For example, they both included in their books the summary of Liu Zi Jue for dispelling diseases and prolonging the life span, which combines controlled breathing with physical exercises, "Open the eyes wide when doing the XU Exercise for the liver. Raise the arms when doing the SI Exercise for the lungs. Hold the head up and cross the hands when doing the HE Exercise for the heart. Keep the knees level when doing the CHUI Exercise for the kidneys. Thrust and round the lips when doing the HU Exercise for the spleen, and lie down when doing the XI Exercise to drive heat from Sanjiao."

There are a number of schools of exercises which incorporate elements of Liu Zi Jue, including Yi Jin Jing (Tendon–Muscle Strengthening Exercises), E Mei Zhuang (Standing Stake Exercises), Xing Yi Quan (12-Animal Shadow Boxing), Ba Gua Zhang (Eight-Diagram Palm) and Da Yan Gong (Wild Goose Exercises). But the sounds are used as an aid to physical exercises in these dynamic Qigong, which is different from Liu Zi Jue. An authoritative work on the subject is Ma Litang's *Liu Zi Jue Health and Fitness Exercises* for clinical application.

The theoretical basis of the Liu Zi Jue exercises is in line with the ancient theories intrinsic to traditional Chinese medicine of the Five Elements (metal, wood, water, fire and earth) and the Five Solid Viscera (heart, liver, spleen, lungs and kidneys). They tend to be on common ground on such issues as mouth forms and pronunciation methods, and the direction of body movements and mind follow the inner circulation law of the meridians of traditional Chinese medicine. Yet, the standardization poses a problem as there have been different points of view on such issues as the pronunciation of the sounds HE and SI, the correct mouth forms and whether the sounds should be pronounced at all, the correspondence between the sounds and the internal organs and the order of these sounds in practice. There are special relationships between the pronunciations and accompanying movements, but they need to be proved by scientific theories and tests. The authors of this book did a lot of research in this respect before compiling this new concept of exercises which are easy to learn and practice.

Chapter II
Characteristics

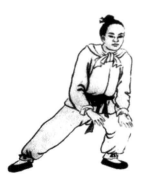

Mouth Forms Required for Pronunciation

Liu Zi Jue features a unique set of special mouth forms to regulate and control the rise and fall of Qi (vital energy) inside the body and related inhalation and exhalation. By means of the breathing and pronunciation methods for XU, HE, HU, SI, CHUI and XI, Liu Zi Jue is unique in balancing the energy and the functions of the inner organs. The authors have tried to standardize the mouth forms and related pronunciation methods, as shown on the accompanying DVD. Such efforts have resulted in a complete system with independent and interactive elements.

Combining Breathing and Movements with Cultivation of Energy

With the focus on breathing and pronouncing the required sounds, Liu Zi Jue features a scientific guideline which helps to regulate the internal organs and enhance the muscles and bones for general health and fitness. Ge Hong of the Eastern Jin Dynasty (317-420) described such effects in a book: "Those who know the real meaning of breathing can enjoy the proper internal circulation of energy vital for the health, and those who know the ways to apply strength and the ways to relax can expect a long life."

Dynamics Infused in Calmness and Flowing Grace

With clear Qigong characteristics, Liu Zi Jue boasts a unique charm of calmness and gentleness, with movements as extended, slow, gentle and graceful as flowing water and clouds. The mysterious and palpable effects are as if one is infused with Qi, leading to a graceful integrity of the body, mind and spirit. The pronunciation is required to be even and extended, and the movements relaxed and slow. Regulated breathing is even required during the inert posture. All this brings one to a calm yet dynamic state, which improves the circulation of vital energy and the functions of the inner organs.

Simple, Reliable and Effective

The exercises are based on the pronunciation of the six sounds during exhalation, accompanied with typical and simple movements. The nine movements, including the ones done in the preparatory and concluding posture, are all easy to learn and practice. The practice requires the mind to follow the circulation of Qi which goes with every stage of the movement, to cultivate the inner energy. Without complicated spiritual striving or difficult, intensive movements, the exercises are safe and reliable, and especially suitable for older people.

Chapter III

Practice Tips

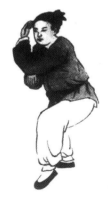

L iu Zi Jue is a set of Qigong exercises for health and fitness, with breathing as the mainstay and simple guiding movements accompanying the breathing routines. Following are recommendations:

Adjusting the Mouth Forms and Feeling the Air Flow

Focus should be placed on correct mouth forms and related air flow when it passes the throat, tongue, teeth and lips. The six mouth forms and related air flow routes have important effects on the vital inner energy and the functions of the inner organs. A correct mouth form is judged from two aspects: the pronunciation and the feeling of the air flow for each of the six sounds.

The beginner can first pronounce the sounds and adjust his or her mouth forms until the correct pronunciation is attained. The practitioner should then try to switch to exhalation with a slight, gentle pronunciation, and finally attain a quiet breathing process.

Combining the Mind with Breathing and Movements

The mind should be in tune with the relaxed, extended movements and even and prolonged breathing and pronunciation. However, excessive concentration is counterproductive. practice should be done in a coordinated and natural manner, and excessive concentration could lead to rigid movements and hurried breathing. The body should be completely relaxed, and excessive effort should be avoided. Only a calm mind and relaxed body can slow the breathing and pulse, so as to set the breathing at an ideal rate. Rigid movements as a result of excessive thought foil the internal balance and functions of the organs. An interactive combination requires the focus to be put on breathing, with the movements as assistants.

Breathing with Slight Control

Breathing consists of natural breathing and the abdominal breathing, and the latter can be divided into direct and reverse breathing. Liu Zi Jue uses reverse breathing, which requires that when the in-breath begins through the nose, the chest cavity should be expanded and the abdomen pulled in. This sequence should be reversed during expiration through the mouth. This increases the upward and downward movements of the diaphragm, effectively massaging the organs, to effectively improve circulation of the blood and vital energy. Beginners should bear in mind that only very slight attention should be paid when breathing, and the breath should be gentle, extended, unconscious and prolonged.

No intentional strength should be applied, and excessive effort to expand or pull in the abdomen is to be avoided at all costs.

Coordinating Breathing with Slow, Relaxed and Gentle Movements

In Liu Zi Jue, breathing is the major practice, accompanied by Qi or vital energy conduction movements which help to flex the joints and enhance the strength and functions of the muscles and bones. The coordination between breathing and pronunciation and the physical exercises should be done in a loose, relaxed, slow and gentle manner to avoid disturbing the even and prolonged breathing and pronunciation.

Step by Step for Consistency

A quiet place with fresh air is most suitable for performing the exercises. A sports suit of loose or other type of comfortable attire helps energy and blood circulation, and makes movement easier. A relaxed body and mind help the practitioner to totally concentrate.

The exercises should be done in a gradual way, and the pace, intensity, length of breathing and times of exercise can be adjusted to suit the health conditions of older people and the weak. After finishing a practice session, it is recommended that one rub the palms and the face, and take a walk to regain the pre-practice status.

Confidence in the effects on health and fitness and perseverance are a must for the exercises to be successful.

Chapter IV

Step-by-Step Descriptions of the Routines

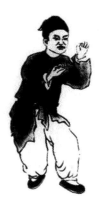

Ready Position

Stand straight, with the feet parallel and shoulder-width apart, and the knees slightly bent. Keep the neck and head erect without straining. Pull in the chin slightly, and contract the chest. Stand straight, with the arms hanging loosely at the sides. Close the mouth, bringing the upper and lower teeth together. Keep the tongue flat, its tip touching lightly the upper palate. Look forward and down. (Fig. 1).

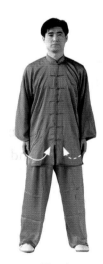

Fig. 1

Key points

- ☐ Breathe naturally through the nose.
- ☐ Keep the mind calm and the body relaxed, with a faint smile.

□ Knees bent not enough or too much, making the hip and knee joints stiff.
□ Thrusting the chest out and looking too far ahead.

□ Keep the knees slightly bent, with the joints relaxed.
□ Pull in the chin, look forward and down, straighten the spine and allow the shoulders to relax forwards slightly.

□ It helps to relax the body and calm the mind, and dredge such meridians as Renmai (or conception vessel, extending along the anterior midline of the body) and Dumai (or governor vessel, extending along the posterior midline of the body) to improve the circulation of the blood and vital energy. Keeps one centered so as to cultivate vital energy, puts the mind at ease and reduces stress.

Starting Position

(*Continue from the previous movement*) Bend the elbows, with the palms up and fingers pointing to each other. Slowly lift the palms to chest level, and look straight ahead. (Figs. 2–3).

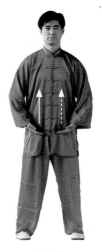
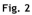

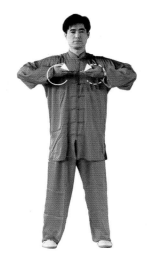

Fig. 2   Fig. 3

Turn the palms inward and downward, and slowly press them down to the level of the navel. Keep the eyes looking straight ahead. (Figs. 4–5).

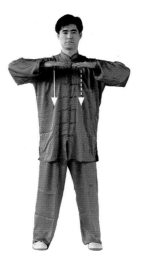

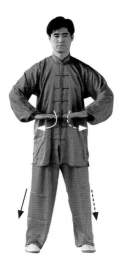

Fig. 4   Fig. 5

Bend the knees slightly, and lower the buttocks. Turn the palms inward and then outward, and slowly push the arms out to form a circle in front of the waist. (Fig. 6).

Turn the palms inward. (Figs. 7 and 7A).

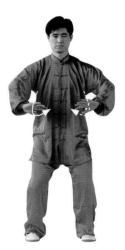

Fig. 6

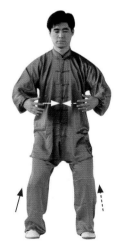

Fig. 7

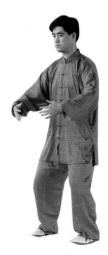

Fig. 7A

Slowly raise the buttocks. Retract the hands and cross their webs between the thumb and the index finger on the navel. Breathe naturally until in a clam frame of mind, while looking forward and down. (Figs. 8 and 8A).

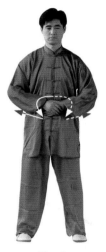

Fig. 8

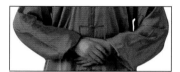

Fig. 8A

Key points

☐ Breathe through the nose.
☐ Inhale while lifting the palms, and exhale when pressing them down and forward. Inhale again when pulling them in.

Common mistakes

☐ Tilting the elbows back and thrusting the chest out while lifting the palms.

- ☐ Thrusting the chest and abdomen out when pushing the palms out.
- ☐ Contracting the elbows and pressing the hands tightly on the navel.

Corrections

- ☐ Move the elbows forward to spread the shoulders and pull in the chest when lifting the palms.
- ☐ Move the body weight backward and stretch the palms forward when pushing the palms out in front of the abdomen.
- ☐ Move the elbows slightly out, and keep the armpits open.

Functions and effects

- ☐ Lifting, pressing down, pushing out and pulling in the hands while rhythmically bending and stretching the lower limbs, accompanied by proper breathing helps to regulate the circulation of inner energy. While vitalizing the blood and energy circulation, it also gets the mind and body ready for the next part of the routine.
- ☐ The rhythmic and gentle movements of the waist and knee joints help to improve and enhance the functions of these joints in middle-aged and older people.

XU Exercise

(嘘字诀)

Routine 1

(*Continue from the previous movement*) Unfold the palms so that they face upward. Touch the little fingers to the waist and slowly draw them back to the sides along the waistline, looking straight ahead. (Fig. 9). Keep the feet in the original position, and turn the upper body a quarter of a turn left-

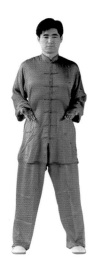

Fig. 9

ward. (Figs. 10 and 10A). Move the right hand slowly forward to shoulder level. Exhale pronouncing the sound "XU" (Shoo). Open the eyes wider to stare fixedly in the direction of the right palm. (Figs. 11 and 11A).

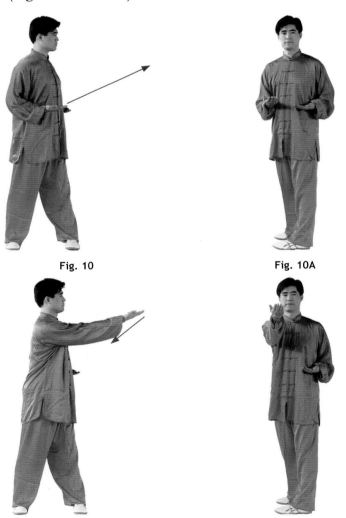

Fig. 10

Fig. 10A

Fig. 11

Fig. 11A

Draw the right hand back to the side of the waist. Turn the upper body a quarter of a turn to face forward. Look forward and down. (Fig. 12).

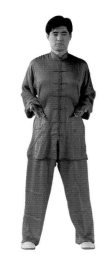

Fig. 12

Turn the upper body a quarter of a turn to the right. (Fig. 13). Move the left palm forward to shoulder level. Exhale, pronouncing the sound "XU." Open the eyes wider to stare fixedly in the direction of the left palm. (Fig. 14).

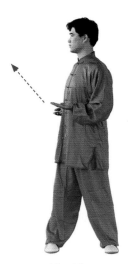

Fig. 13

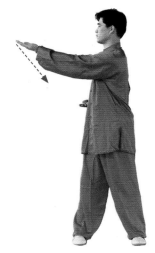

Fig. 14

Draw the left hand back to the side of the waist. Turn the upper body a quarter of a turn to face forward. Look forward and down. (Fig. 15).

Repeat the above movements three times to the left and right, exhaling and pronouncing the sound "XU" six times.

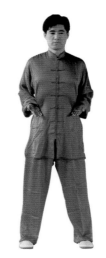

Fig. 15

Key points

☐ The pronunciation is assisted by the teeth. The upper and lower teeth should be parallel with each other, leaving a gap between the teeth and the tongue. Air is exhaled from the gaps between the teeth and between the teeth and the tongue, with the corners of the mouth drawn backward a little. (Fig. 16).

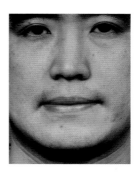

Fig. 16

☐ Exhale pronouncing "XU" while moving the hand forward, and inhale through the nose while drawing the hand back. Close coordination is required between the body movements and the breathing.

Common mistakes

☐ Lack of coordination between body movements and breathing.
☐ Hand moving in the wrong direction.

□ The center of body weight is moved either forward, back-ward or sideways when turning the upper body.

Corrections

□ Synchronizing exhalation and moving the hand forward so that when the latter is completed, the breathing is finished.
□ The fingers should point to the left or right side when the hands are moved in these directions.
□ Keep the feet rooted flat on the floor and turn the upper body around the body's vertical axis.

Functions and effects

□ The theory of traditional Chinese medicine holds that the liver will respond when "XU" is pronounced, and that exhalation and the pronunciation of "XU" help to clear the organ of turbid Qi and regulate its function. Making the eyes glare helps dredge the channels inside the liver and improve the eyesight.

□ Moving the hands right and left alternately helps to promote the functional activities of the liver and improve the circulation of the blood and internal energy.
□ Turning the upper body exercises the organs in the waist and abdomen. It also improves the functions of the waist, knees and digestion of middle-aged and older people, and dredges and regulates the Daimai meridian (belt vessel) or the channel around the waist, as well as the circulation of energy inside the body as a whole.

HE Exercise

(呵字诀)

Routine 2

1. (*Continue from the previous routine as shown in Fig. 15*) Inhale and at the same time slightly lift the hands with the little fingers touching the sides of the waist and the fingers tilted forward and down. Look straight ahead. (Fig. 17). Bend the knees to squat down, lower the hands downward to about 45 degrees, and move forward with the arms slightly bent and the eyes fixed on the hands. (Figs. 18 and 18A).

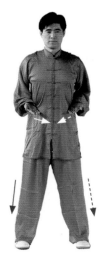

Fig. 17

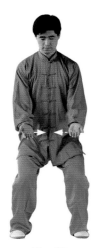

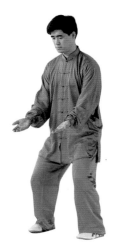

Fig. 18　　　　　　　　　　**Fig. 18A**

2. Slightly bend the elbows and draw the hands back. The little fingers should be touching each other, and the palms should be up in a hollow lifting position level with the navel. Fix the eyes on the hands. (Figs. 19 and 19A).

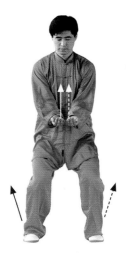

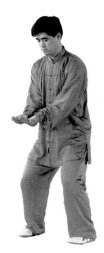

Fig. 19　　　　　　　　　　**Fig. 19A**

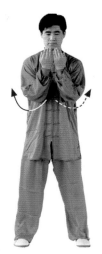

Fig. 20

3. Slowly straighten the knees to stand up, bend the elbows and lift the hands to chest level, with the palms facing the chest and the middle fingers level with the chin. Look forward and down. (Figs. 20 and 20A).

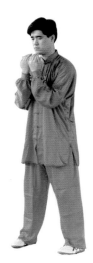

Fig. 20A

4. Lift the elbows outward and level with the shoulders. Turn the palms down, with the fingers pointing down and the backs of the hands touching each other. (Figs. 21 and 21A). Lower the hands and look forward and down. (Figs. 22 and 22A). Exhale to pronounce "HE" (Her) while lowering the hands.

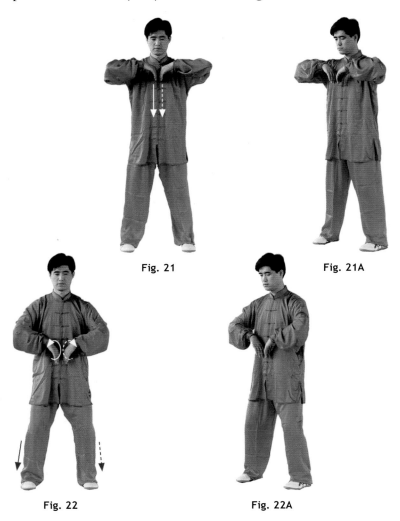

Fig. 21

Fig. 21A

Fig. 22

Fig. 22A

5. Bend the knees to slightly squat down while moving the palms down to a position level with the navel. Turn the palms down and out, and push them slowly out to form a circle. Look forward and down. (Fig. 23).

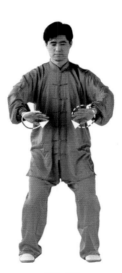

Fig. 23

6. Turn the palms inward and then up, and draw the elbows inward to form a hollow lifting position in front of the abdomen. Look at the palms. (Figs. 24, 25 and 26).

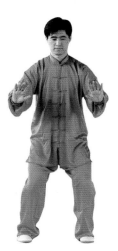

Fig. 24

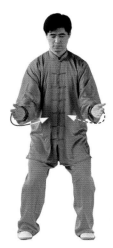

Fig. 25

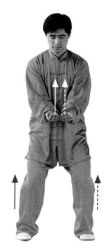

Fig. 26

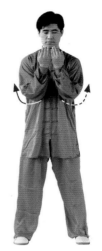

Fig. 27

7. Slowly straighten the knees to stand up. Bend the elbows to lift the hands to chest level, with the palms facing the chest and the middle fingers level with the chin. Look forward and down. (Figs. 27 and 27A).

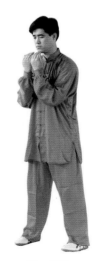

Fig. 27A

8. Lift the elbows outward and up to shoulder level. Turn the palms down, with the fingers pointing down and the backs of the hands touching each other. (Figs. 28 and 28A). Lower the hands, and look forward and down. (Figs. 29 and 29A). Exhale to pronounce "HE" while lowering the hands.

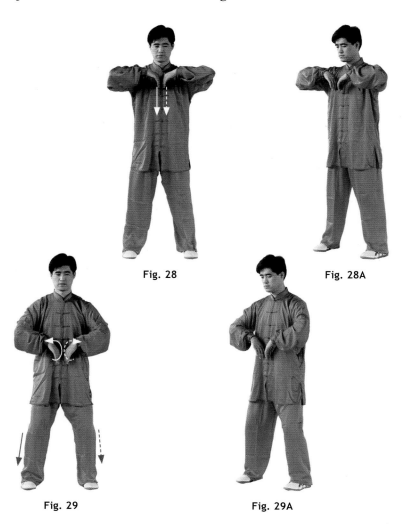

Fig. 28

Fig. 28A

Fig. 29

Fig. 29A

Repeat movements 5 to 8 four times, pronouncing "HE" six times in the process.

Key points

□ The pronunciation of "HE" is assisted by the tongue. When exhaling and pronouncing the sound, touch the upper back teeth lightly with the sides of the tongue and exhale the air from between the tongue and the upper jaw. (Fig. 30).

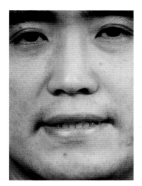

Fig. 30

□ Inhale through the nose when lifting the hands, and exhale and pronounce "HE" when moving the hands down and pushing them out.

Common mistakes

□ Thrusting the chest out and the head up when lifting the hands and bending the elbows.

Corrections

□ Keep the head down and pull in the chest when bending the elbows.

Functions and effects

☐ The theory of traditional Chinese medicine holds that the heart will respond when the sound "HE" is pronounced, and that exhalation while pronouncing "HE" will help to rid the heart of turbid Qi and regulate its function.

☐ The raising and lowering of the hands help to promote the function of the kidneys, which correspond to water according to traditional Chinese medicine. The water then will help to expel fire from the heart, which will go down to warm the water in the kidneys. Such an interaction regulates and invigorates the functions of both the heart and kidneys.

☐ The gentle and continuous exercising of the hands, shoulders, elbows and wrists and related joints improves their flexibility and coordination, thus helping to prevent degeneration of the joints of the upper body in older and middle-aged people.

HU Exercise

(呼字诀)

Routine 3

1. After pushing out the hands. (Fig. 31) in the last routine, turn the palms inward to face the navel, with the fingers apart and tilted towards each other, and the palms apart as far from the navel as from each other. Look forward and down. (Fig. 32).

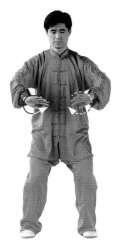

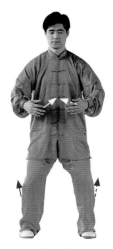

Fig. 31   Fig. 32

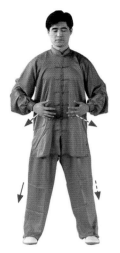

Fig. 33

2. Slowly straighten the knees to stand up, and slowly move the hands together to a position some 10 cm in front of the navel. (Fig. 33).

3. Slightly squat down, and at the same time, move the hands out as far from the navel as from each other to form a circle. Pronounce "HU" (Hoo), looking forward and down. (Figs. 34 and 34A).

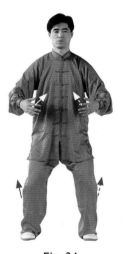

Fig. 34

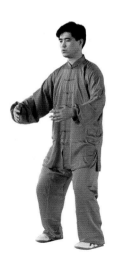

Fig. 34A

4. Slowly straighten the knees to stand up, at the same time bringing the palms slowly towards the navel. (Fig. 35).

Repeat movements 3 to 4 five times, pronouncing "HU" six times in the process.

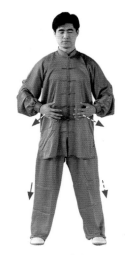

Fig. 35

Key points

- The pronunciation of "HU" is assisted by the throat. In the process of exhalation and pronunciation, curve the sides of the tongue up, thrust the lips forward to form a round opening, and exhale through the opening. (Fig. 36).
- Inhale while moving the hands closer to the navel, and exhale to pronounce "HU" when moving the hands out.

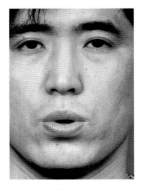

Fig. 36

- ☐ Thrusting the waist and abdomen out when extending the hands.
- ☐ Knees buckle inwards or bow outwards.

Corrections

- ☐ Lower the hips, move the body weight backward and apply strength to the hands and arms when extending them, with the waist and hands moving in opposite directions.
- ☐ Keep knees pointing in the same direction as the feet.

Functions and effects

- ☐ The theory of traditional Chinese medicine holds that the spleen will respond when the sound "HU" is pronounced, and that the exhalation and pronunciation of "HU" help to rid the spleen and stomach of turbid Qi and regulate their functions.

- ☐ Moving the hands close to and away from the navel helps to refresh the internal circulation, contraction and extension 0 of the abdominal cavity. It helps to massage the intestines and stomach, strengthens the spleen and stomach, and helps to cure indigestion.

SI Exercise

(呬字诀)

Routine 4

1. (*Continue from the previous movement, as in Fig. 34*) Lower the hands with the palms facing up, and point the fingers at each other. Look forward and down. (Fig. 37).

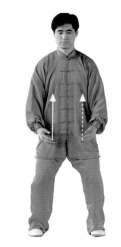

Fig. 37

2. Slowly straighten the knees to stand up. Raise the hands to chest level. Look forward and down. (Fig. 38).

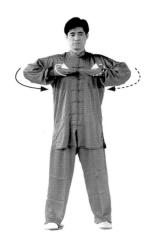

Fig. 38

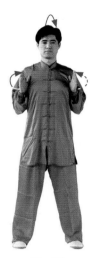

Fig. 39

3. Lower the elbows, and draw them back to the flanks. Raise the hands to shoulder height, with the fingers pointing up. (Figs. 39 and 39A).

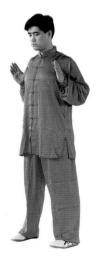

Fig. 39A

Pull in the shoulder blades towards the spine by spreading the shoulders and the chest. Tilt the head back a little while pulling in the neck. Look forward and up. (Figs. 40, 40A and 40B).

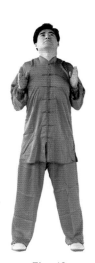

Fig. 40

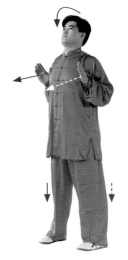

Fig. 40A

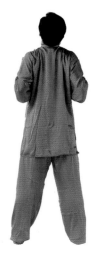

Fig. 40B

4. Adopt a slight squatting position, at the same time relaxing the shoulders and making the neck straight. Slowly push the palms forward while pronouncing "SI" (Tser). Keep the eyes fixed straight ahead. (Figs. 41 and 42).

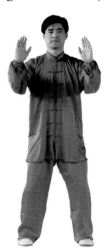

Fig. 41

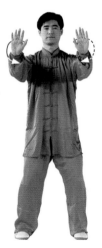

Fig. 42

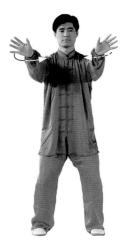

Fig. 43

5. Turn the wrists in an outward circle to face the palms inward, with the fingers pointing to each other and shoulder-width apart. (Figs. 43 and 44).

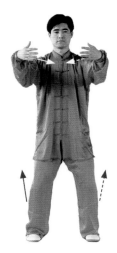

Fig. 44

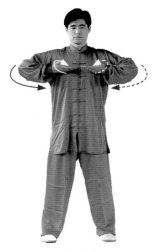

Fig. 45

6. Slowly straighten the knees to stand up, at the same time bending the elbows and slowly withdrawing the hands to a position about 10 cm in front of the chest, with the palms up and fingers pointing to each other. Look forward and down. (Fig. 45).

7. Lower the elbows, and make them touch the ribs. Raise the hands to shoulder height, with the palms facing each other and the fingers pointing up. (Figs. 46 and 46A). Pull in the shoulder blades

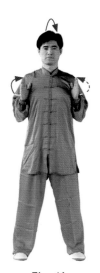

Fig. 46

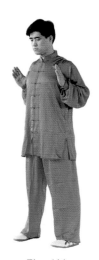

Fig. 46A

towards the spine. Spread the shoulders and chest. Pull in the neck while tilting the head back a little, and look forward and up. (Figs. 47, 47A and 47B).

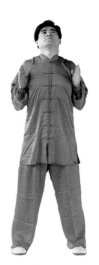

Fig. 47

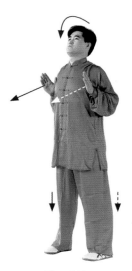

Fig. 47A

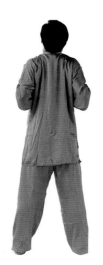

Fig. 47B

8. Adopt a slight squatting position, at the same time relaxing the shoulders and keeping the neck straight. Slowly extend the hands forward while pronouncing "SI," palms facing forward. Keep the eyes fixed straight ahead. (Figs. 48 and 49).

Repeat movements 5 to 8 four times, pronouncing "SI" a total of six times.

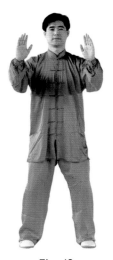

Fig. 48

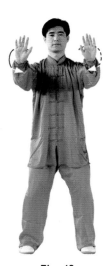

Fig. 49

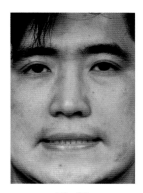

Fig.50

□ The pronunciation of "SI" is assisted by the teeth. In the process of exhalation and pronunciation, make the front upper and lower teeth parallel, with a narrow gap in between. The tongue tip touches lightly the lower teeth. Exhale the air from between the teeth. (Fig. 50).

□ Exhale and pronounce "SI" while pushing the hands out. Turn the wrists outward, with the fingers pointing to each other. Inhale through the nose when withdrawing the hands.

Common mistakes

□ Complete the acts of raising the palms, spreading the shoulders and the chest, tilting the head back a little to pull in the neck at the same point in time. Moving the head backward too much when pulling in the neck.

55

Corrections

□ Raise the hands to shoulder level; then spread the shoulders and chest; and then tilt the head back a little to pull in the neck. These movements should be done step by step.
□ When tilting the head back and pulling in the neck, pull in the chin slightly.

Functions and effects

☐ The theory of traditional Chinese medicine holds that the lungs will respond when the sound "SI" is pronounced, and that the exhalation and the pronunciation of "SI" help to rid the lungs of turbid Qi and regulate its function.

☐ Spreading the shoulders and chest, and pulling in the neck by somewhat tilting the head back help to fill the lung cavities with fresh air. Contracting the lower abdomen raises internal energy from Dantian (about two inches below the navel) upward to the chest. The convergence in the chest of fresh air and energy helps to improve the breathing, thus invigorating the refreshment of Qi and blood and air exchange in the lungs.

☐ Raising the hands to shoulder height, relaxing the shoulders and pushing the hands forward stimulate the points around the shoulders, effectively reducing muscle and joint fatigue at the shoulders, neck and back, and preventing cervical problems, periarthritis and back muscle fatigue.

CHUI Exercise

(吹字诀)

Routine 5

1. (*Continue from the previous routine as in Fig. 49*) Extend the hands, relax the wrists and point the fingers forward, with the palms down. (Fig. 51).

2. Move the arms apart and hold them level with the shoulders, with the palms tilted backward and fingers pointing outward. (Fig. 52).

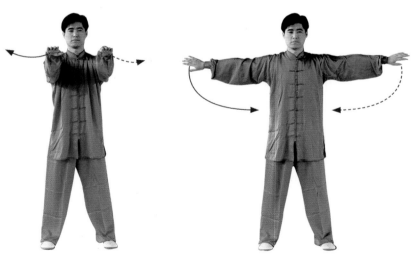

Fig. 51   Fig. 52

3. Turn the arms inward. Move the palms in a curve to the back of the waist, with the palms gently touching the Yaoyan points on the back near the spine and the fingers tilted down. Look forward and down. (Figs. 53, 53A, 54 and 54A).

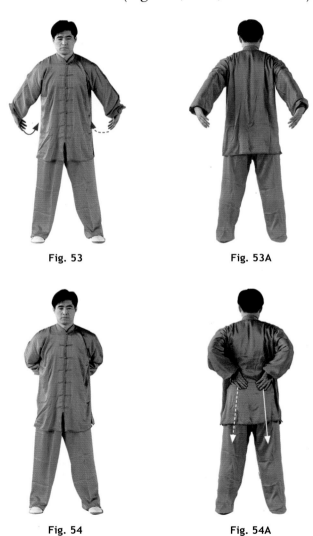

Fig. 53   Fig. 53A

Fig. 54   Fig. 54A

4. Slightly bend the knees to squat down, at the same time moving the palms down along the back of the waist, hips and thighs. Bend the elbows to lift the arms from the back of the body to the front for a hollow holding position in front of the navel, with the palms facing inward and fingers pointing towards each other. Look forward and down. (Figs. 55, 55A, 56, 56A and 57). Exhale to pronounce "CHUI" (Chway) when moving the hands down from the back of the waist.

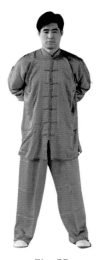

Fig. 55

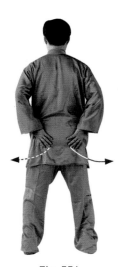

Fig. 55A

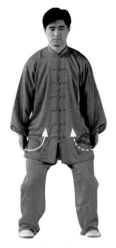

Fig. 56

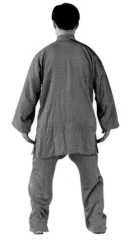

Fig. 56A

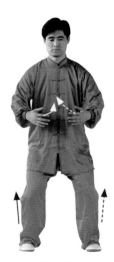

Fig. 57

5. Slowly straighten the knees to stand up, and at the same time draw the palms back to gently touch the abdomen, with the fingers tilted down at an angle and the thumbs pointing towards each other. Look forward and down. (Fig. 58).

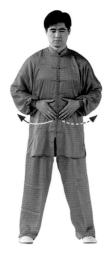

Fig. 58

6. Move the hands backward along the waist. (Fig. 59).

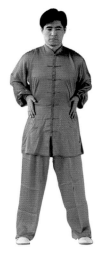

Fig. 59

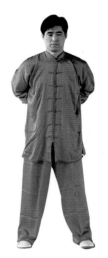

Fig. 60

7. Move the hands to the back of the waist, with the palms slightly touching the Yaoyan points on the back of the waist near the spine and with fingers pointing down at an angle. Look forward and down. (Fig. 60 and 60A).

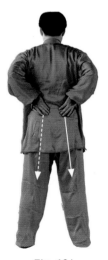

Fig. 60A

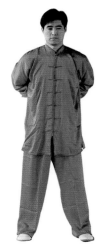

Fig. 61

8. Slightly bend the knees to squat down, and at the same time move the hands along and down the back of the waist, hips and thighs. Bend the elbows to lift the arms from the back of the body to the front for a hollow holding position in front of the navel, with the palms facing inward and the fingers pointing to each other. Look forward and down. (Figs. 61, 61A, 62 and 62A and 63).

Repeat movements 5 to 8 four times, pronouncing "CHUI" a total of six times.

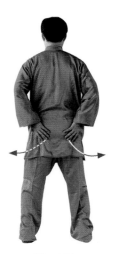

Fig. 61A

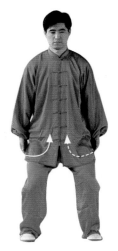

Fig. 62

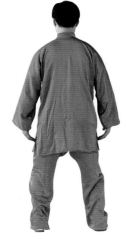

Fig. 62A

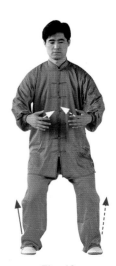

Fig. 63

☐ The pronunciation of "CHUI" is assisted by the lips. In the process of exhalation and pronunciation, pull back the tongue and the corners of the mouth, make the back teeth parallel, draw the lips back to a stretched state, and exhale the air from the throat through the sides of the tongue and between the stretched lips. (Fig. 64).

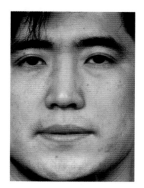

Fig.64

☐ Exhale and pronounce "CHUI" when moving the hands down the back of the waist and lifting them to a hollow holding position in front of the abdomen. Inhale through the nose when moving the hands backward along the waist.

Common mistakes

☐ The movements are stiff when bending the knees to squat down and moving the hands down along the back of the waist and thighs.

Corrections

☐ Relax the arms and body to feel the motion of the falling palms.

65

Functions and effects

□ The theory of traditional Chinese medicine holds that the kidneys will respond when the sound "CHUI" is pronounced, and that the exhalation and pronunciation of "CHUI" helps to get rid of turbid Qi in the kidneys and to regulate their function.

□ The theory holds that the waist is the home of the kidneys. As they are located on the sides of the spine, the function of the waist is closely linked with the functional activities of the kidneys. Hand-massage of the waist and abdomen strengthens the waist and kidneys, improves their functions, and prevents aging.

XI Exercise

(嘻字诀)

Routine 6

1. (*Continue from the previous routine, as in Fig. 63*) Move the hands down from the hollow holding position to in front of the lower abdomen. Look forward and down. (Fig. 65), turn the palms inward and out, with the backs of the hands close to each other, the palms facing out and the fingers pointing down. Look at the hands. (Fig. 66).

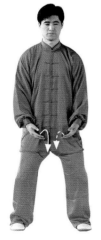

Fig. 65

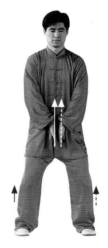

Fig. 66

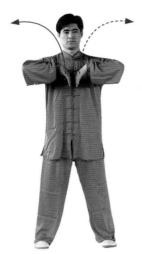

Fig. 67

2. Slowly straighten the knees to stand up, lift the elbows and the hands to a position in front of the chest. (Fig. 67).

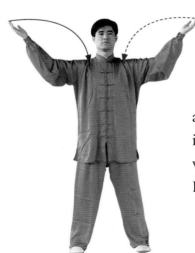

Fig. 68

Raise the hands to face height and curve them outward to a holding position distant from the head, with the palms angled upward. Look forward and up. (Fig. 68).

3. Bend the elbows to draw the hands back to a position in front of the chest and level with the shoulders, with the fingers pointing at each other and the palms down. Look forward and down. (Fig. 69).

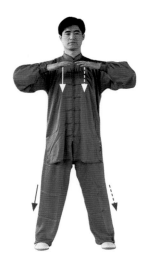

Fig. 69

Slightly bend the knees to assume a squatting position, at the same time slowly lowering the hands to a position in front of the navel. (Fig. 70).

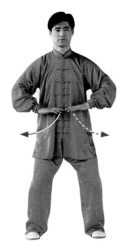

Fig. 70

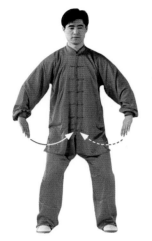

Fig. 71

4. Continue to lower and separate the hands, until they are in a position about 15 cm from the sides of the hip-bones, with the palms facing outward and fingers pointing down. Look forward and down. (Fig. 71). Exhale and start to pronounce the sound "XI" (Shee) when lowering the hands.

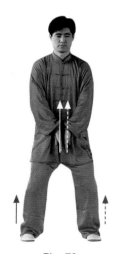

Fig. 72

5. Bring the hands to a position in front of the lower abdomen, with the palms facing outward and the fingers pointing down. Fix the eyes on the hands. (Fig. 72).

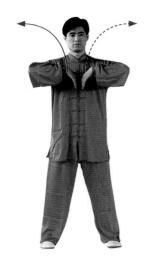

Fig. 73

6. Slowly straighten the knees to stand up, lift the elbows and the hands to a position in front of the chest. (Fig. 73).

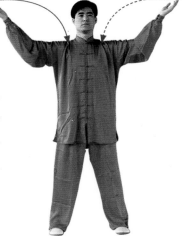

Fig. 74

Raise the hands to face level, and then curve them outward to a holding position distant from the head, with the palms angled upward. Look forward and up. (Fig. 74).

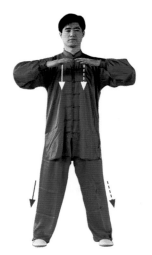

Fig. 75

7. Bend the elbows to draw the hands back to a position in front of the chest and level with the shoulders, with the fingers pointing towards each other and the palms down. Look forward and down. (Fig. 75).

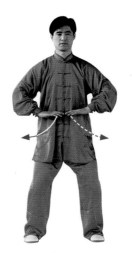

Fig. 76

Slightly bend the knees to assume a squatting position, at the same time slowly lowering the hands to a position in front of the navel. Look forward and down. (Fig. 76).

8. Continue to press the hands down and out to a position about 15 cm from the sides of the hipbones, with the palms facing outward and the fingers pointing down. Look forward and down. (Fig. 77). Exhale, and start to pronounce the sound "XI" when lowering the hands.

Repeat movements 5 to 8 four times, pronouncing "Xi" a total of six times.

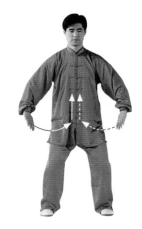

Fig. 77

Key points

☐ The pronunciation of "XI" is assisted by the teeth. In the process of exhalation and pronunciation, touch the lower teeth with the tip of the tongue, draw the corners of the mouth slightly back and up, slightly close the back teeth, and exhale through the gap between the back teeth. (Fig. 78).

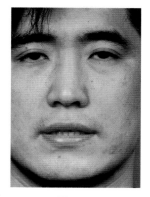

Fig. 78

- Inhale through the nose when lifting the elbows, separating and lifting the hands. Exhale to pronounce "XI" when pressing the hands down and out in a relaxed manner.

Common mistakes

- Straightening the knees to stand up when lowering the hands from the hollow holding position in the previous movement to a position in front of the lower abdomen.

Corrections

- Keep the knees bent at the correct angle when lowering the hands.

Functions and effects

- The theory of traditional Chinese medicine holds that the vital energy from the Shaoyang meridian and from the Shanjiao (three portions of the body cavities housing the internal organs) will respond when the sound "XI" is pronounced, and that the exhalation and pronunciation of "XI" help to dredge the channels and improve internal energy circulation and the functions of various organs.
- The series of movements such as raising, separating, extending or pressing down, relaxing, turning in, and bringing the hands together help to expand or contract the breathing cavities. The two functions are interactive and jointly regulate blood and energy circulation throughout the body.

Closing Form

(*Continue from the previous movement, as in Fig. 77*) Turn the palms inward (Fig. 79), slowly move them to the front of the abdomen and place one over the other by crossing their webs between the thumb and the index finger to slightly cover the navel. At the same time, slowly straighten the knees to stand up. Look forward and down. (Figs. 80 and 81).

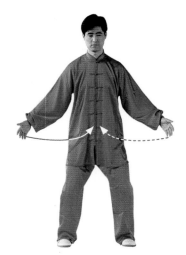

Fig. 79

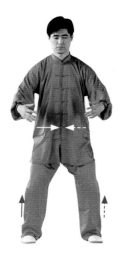

Fig. 80

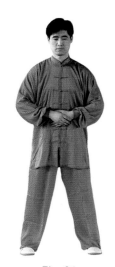

Fig. 81

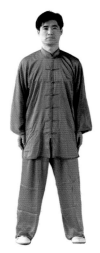

Rub the abdomen around the navel, first six circles clockwise and then another six circles anticlockwise.

Let the hands hang loosely at the sides. Look forward and down. (Fig. 82).

Fig. 82

Key points

☐ Relax the body to ensure a calm mind, with Qi collected and regulated to preserve quiet internal cultivation.

Functions and effects

☐ Qi collection and regulation and rubbing the abdomen around the navel help to conduct the vital energy back to its original location, and help the practitioner to regain the preexercise state.

Appendix

Acupuncture Points
Mentioned in This Book

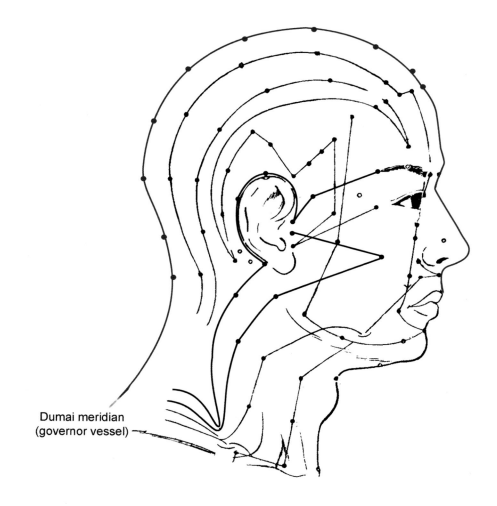

Dumai meridian
(governor vessel)

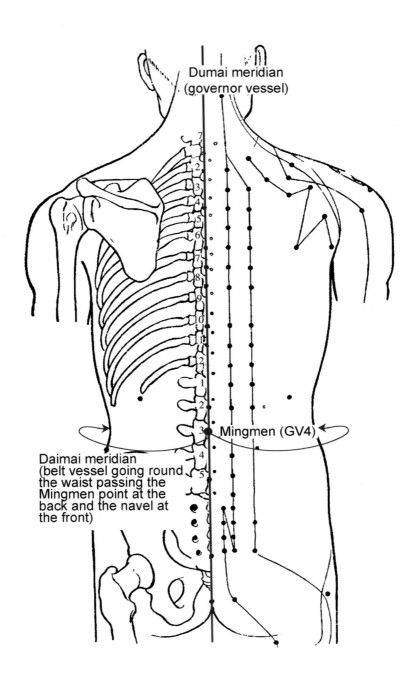

Dumai meridian
(governor vessel)

Mingmen (GV4)

Daimai meridian
(belt vessel going round
the waist passing the
Mingmen point at the
back and the navel at
the front)